The Acne-Free Diet Plan Cook Book

Maintaining a Healthy Diet Free of Acne: Important Facts and Delicious Recipes

REX LEWIS

Table of Contents

Introduction **5**

CHAPTER ONE **11**

The Relationship Between Acne and Diet..................................**11**

An Overview of Acne **17**

CHAPTER TWO............................**24**

Variety of Acne **24**

Triggers and Causes **29**

CHAPTER THREE **36**

How Diet Impacts Acne................**36**

CHAPTER FOUR............................**43**

Nutrients for Clear Skin...............**43**

Antioxidants and Their Role.......**49**

Minerals for Acne Prevention **56**

CHAPTER FIVE..............................**62**

Foods to Include for Clear Skin..**62**

Foods to Avoid for Acne-Free Skin **68**

Prominent Causes of Acne Outbreaks 75

CHAPTER SIX 82

Developing a Meal Plan for Clear Skin 82

Optimizing Nutrient Balance for Optimal Impact 89

CHAPTER SEVEN 96

Habits of Lifestyle for Clear Skin 96

The Value of Consistent Exercise 103

Methods to Achieve Clear Skin 111

Supplements to Heal Acne 117

Conclusion 124

THE END 129

Introduction

Common skin condition acne is caused by the clogging of hair follicles with dead skin cells and sebum. It frequently results in the development of blackheads, whiteheads, acne, and occasionally deeper lesions or nodules. Acne predominantly impacts regions of the skin that contain an abundance of oil glands, including the face, chest, back, and shoulders.

The following are significant contributing factors to the onset of acne:

Sebum Production in Excess: Sebaceous glands located in the epidermis generate a viscous substance known as sebum. Acne can result when an excess of sebum produced by these glands combines with decaying skin cells to obstruct hair follicles.

Clogging of Hair Follicles: When dead skin cells combine with sebum, they can accumulate and form a blockage that obstructs hair follicles. This setting is particularly conducive to the proliferation of bacteria.

Bacteria (Propionibacterium acnes): Typically found on the skin,

P. acnes can proliferate and contribute to inflammation and the development of acne when hair follicles become obstructed.

Hormonal fluctuations, which are prevalent during specific medical conditions, menstruation, pregnancy, and puberty, can stimulate sebaceous glands to increase oil production. This increased oil secretion has the potential to exacerbate acne.

A family history of acne may contribute to an increased susceptibility to the condition. The susceptibility of the epidermis to inflammation and its response to hormones can both be influenced by genetic factors.

Diet and Lifestyle: Although the precise influence of diet on acne remains uncertain, several research studies indicate that specific foods, including dairy and carbohydrates with a high glycemic index, might worsen the condition in some individuals. Stress and sleep deprivation may also contribute to the issue.

Environmental factors: Proximity to specific environmental elements, including pollution and humidity, may either initiate the progression of acne or worsen preexisting conditions.

Acne may be categorized into the following classifications:

A whitehead is a clogged or closed pore.

Blackheads: Open, clogged pores; the pigmentation is caused by oxidized melanin and not grime.

Pupils are delicate, reddish-pimples.

Pustules are pus-filled pustules.

Nodules are excruciating, sizable masses located beneath the skin's surface.

Cysts are excruciating, deep, pus-filled nodules.

Acne treatment strategies differ based on the severity of the condition, but may involve oral or topical medications, modifications to one's lifestyle, and, in extreme cases, medical interventions. It is recommended that individuals seek the expertise of a dermatologist in order to receive customized recommendations and treatment alternatives that are tailored to their specific skin requirements.

CHAPTER ONE
The Relationship Between Acne and Diet

Ongoing research investigates the correlation between diet and acne. Although not entirely conclusive, there exists evidence indicating that specific dietary components might impact the onset or worsening of acne. It is essential to note, however, that individual responses to diet can vary, and the impacts will not be identical for everyone. A number of factors warrant consideration:

• Acne may be exacerbated by a diet rich in refined carbohydrates and foods with a high glycemic index (GI), according to some studies. Elevated glycemic index (GI) foods have the potential to induce a surge in insulin levels, subsequently impeding sebum (oil) production and potentially exacerbating acne progression. High-GI foods include items such as white bread, sugary treats, and sweetened beverages.

• **Dairy Products:** Some evidence suggests that dairy product consumption is associated with an increased risk of acne. The potential impact of specific milk components, including hormones and growth factors, on skin health has been postulated. Specifically, skim milk has been linked to an increased risk in comparison to whole milk.

• An inflammation-inducing dietary disparity between omega-6 and omega-3 fatty acids may potentially play a role in the development of acne. In comparison to omega-3 fatty acids, which are found in fish and specific seeds, Western diets are generally more abundant in omega-6 fatty acids, which are found in vegetable oils.

• There has been ongoing debate regarding the correlation between the consumption of chocolate and acne. Although some studies indicate a potential correlation, further investigation is required to definitively establish a link.

• Acne may potentially be attributed to nutrient deficiencies, specifically in zinc and antioxidants such as vitamin E and vitamin A. These nutrients must be consumed in sufficient quantities to promote overall skin health.

• Caution should be exercised when considering the correlation between diet and acne, given the ongoing nature of research in this field and the inconsistent findings that have been reported in some studies. Furthermore, variations in individual reactions to dietary modifications may occur. If you suspect that your acne may be influenced by your diet, take into account the following:

• Maintain a food journal to track your dietary intake and identify any recurring trends that may indicate a connection between particular foods and acne outbreaks.

It is advisable to implement dietary changes in a gradual manner. Unpredictable alterations might fail to offer definitive insights into the consequences for one's skin.

Seeking Professional Advice: For personalized guidance regarding concerns regarding the correlation between your diet and acne, it is advisable to consult with a dermatologist or other healthcare professional.

In conclusion, for optimal skin health, it is critical to adhere to proper skincare practices, consume a well-balanced diet, and stay hydrated. Consultation with a healthcare professional is advisable in the case of persistent acne, in order to obtain an accurate diagnosis and develop an appropriate treatment regimen.

An Overview of Acne

A common skin condition, acne is caused by the clogging of hair follicles with dead skin cells, oil, and occasionally bacteria. The condition is distinguished by the development of a diverse array of skin lesions, such as blackheads, whiteheads, acne, and in more advanced instances, cysts or nodules. A brief overview of acne:

1. Follicles of hair and sebaceous glands:

• Acne predominantly impacts regions of the skin that contain an abundance of oil glands, including the face, chest, back, and shoulders.

• Sebaceous glands are responsible for the production of sebum, an oily substance that lubricates the skin.

2. Development of Acne Lesions:

• Whiteheads (Closed Comedones): A combination of dead skin cells and oil clogs pores, producing a closed, small bump.

• Blackheads, which are open comedones, resemble whiteheads but are darker in appearance. Their dark hue is caused by the oxidation of melanin rather than dirt.

- Papules are raised, reddish bumps that develop as a result of infection and inflammation within clogged hair follicles.

- Pustules are pus-filled zits distinguished by a yellow or white center.

Nodules and cysts are deep-seated, more severe lesions that may cause pain and result in the formation of scar tissue.

3. Bacterial Participation:

- On the skin, the bacterium Propionibacterium acnes (P. acnes) is present.

P. acnes can proliferate when hair follicles become obstructed, resulting in inflammation and the development of acne lesions.

4. Aspects of hormonal influence:

- Specifically during puberty, menstruation, pregnancy, and specific medical conditions, hormonal fluctuations can stimulate sebaceous glands to generate additional oil.

An elevated production of oil may be a factor in the onset of acne.

5. Contributing Genetic Factors:

• A history of acne in the family may heighten susceptibility.

Hormones and inflammation can induce distinct skin responses that are influenced by genetic factors.

6. Lifestyle and Environmental Factors:

• Acne can be influenced by environmental factors such as pollution and humidity.

• Additionally, stress and insufficient sleep may contribute to the worsening of acne.

7. Variety of Acne:

Manifestations of mild acne include blackheads and whiteheads.

Included in moderate acne are pustules and papules.

Scarring-causing nodules and cysts are characteristics of severe acne.

8. Treatment Methods:

• Depending on the severity of the condition, treatment may consist of oral medications (e.g., oral contraceptives, retinoids, benzoyl peroxide), topical medications (e.g., benzoyl peroxide), or laser therapy or chemical peels in extreme cases.

It is essential to engage in skin care routines, including gentle cleansing and avoiding vigorous scrubbing.

Noting that acne is a prevalent and treatable condition is essential. A consultation with a dermatologist can assist in determining the most effective treatment for acne, taking into consideration the individual's skin type and condition.

CHAPTER TWO
Variety of Acne

Acne exhibits a diverse array of manifestations, with the condition varying in severity from mild to severe. The following are frequent forms of acne lesions:

Whiteheads, also known as closed comedones, are:

Small, closed bumps on the surface of the skin.

Coats the pores with a combination of dead skin cells and oil.

The pore aperture is sealed, thereby impeding air exposure.

Comedones that are outwardly blackheads:

Comparable to whiteheads, but with an exposed pore on the surface of the skin.

The darkness is not the result of dirt, but rather the oxidation of melanin.

Papules, or Tiny, elevated, red bumps.

Caused by infection and inflammation of clogged hair follicles.

Not generally filled with pus.

- **Ostioleal pustules:**

Pimples containing pus at their white or yellow center.

A red base with a visible pus-filled center.

Possible tenderness upon contact.

Nodules consist of:

Solid, painful, larger nodules located beneath the skin's surface.

When the contents of a pustule or papule penetrate more deeply into the skin, they develop.

Potentially scarring.

Cysts, or:

Deep, excruciating, pus-filled nodules.

More enormous and severe in size than pustules and nodules.

Potential for scarring.

These distinct varieties of acne lesions may manifest singly or in clusters. Although "comedones" encompasses both blackheads and whiteheads, the remaining categories pertain to inflammatory reactions. Although acne lesions can manifest on other body parts, the face, chest, back, and shoulders are the most common locations.

Frequently, acne is classified according to its severity:

Mild acne is distinguished by the existence of both blackheads and whiteheads.

Indicators of moderate acne are pustules and papules.

Severe acne manifests as cysts and nodules, which may result in more extensive scarring.

In severe cases, medical procedures may be necessary in addition to topical treatments, oral medications, and lifestyle modifications in order to effectively manage acne. A consultation with a dermatologist, who can assess the severity and nature of acne in order to determine the most effective course of treatment, can be beneficial.

Triggers and Causes

Multiple factors contribute to the initiation and progression of acne, encompassing genetic, hormonal, environmental, and lifestyle elements. The leading causes and triggers of acne are as follows:

1. Hormonal Variations:

• Hormonal fluctuations, especially during puberty, menstruation, pregnancy, and conditions like polycystic ovary syndrome (PCOS), can lead to increased sebum (oil) production.

•   Elevated androgen levels stimulate the sebaceous glands, contributing to the development of acne.

2. Excess Sebum Production:

• Sebaceous glands produce an oily substance called sebum to lubricate the skin.

• Overproduction of sebum can lead to clogged pores and the formation of acne lesions.

3. Hair Follicle Clogging:

• Dead skin cells can accumulate and mix with sebum, forming plugs that block hair follicles.

• This creates an environment conducive to bacterial growth, particularly Propionibacterium acnes (P. acnes).

4. Bacterial Infection (P. acnes):

• P. acnes is a bacterium normally present on the skin.

• When hair follicles are blocked, P. acnes can multiply, leading to inflammation and the development of acne lesions.

5. Genetics:

• A family history of acne may increase an individual's susceptibility.

• Hormones and inflammation can induce distinct skin responses that are influenced by genetic factors.

6. Diet:

• While the link between diet and acne is not fully understood, some studies suggest that certain factors may contribute, such as a high-glycemic diet (refined carbohydrates) and dairy products.

More research is needed to establish clear connections between specific foods and acne.

7. Environmental Factors:

• Exposure to pollutants, high humidity, and certain climates may influence acne.

• Prolonged exposure to environmental factors can affect the skin's health and exacerbate existing acne conditions.

8. Stress:

• Stress may contribute to the development or worsening of acne through various mechanisms, including hormonal fluctuations and increased sebum production.

9. Medications:

- Certain medications, such as corticosteroids, and some hormonal medications, can contribute to acne development.

- Always consult with healthcare professionals about potential side effects of medications.

10. Cosmetics and Skincare Products:

- Some cosmetics and skincare products may contain ingredients that can clog pores and contribute to acne.

Using non-comedogenic products can help prevent pore blockage.

Understanding the underlying causes and triggers of acne is crucial for effective management. Treatment approaches often involve a combination of topical treatments, oral medications, lifestyle modifications, and skincare practices. If acne is persistent or severe, seeking guidance from a dermatologist is advisable to develop a personalized treatment plan.

CHAPTER THREE
How Diet Impacts Acne

The relationship between diet and acne is a complex and evolving area of research. While the exact mechanisms are not fully understood, some studies suggest that certain dietary factors may influence the development or exacerbation of acne in some individuals. Here are some ways in which diet may impact acne:

High-Glycemic Diet:

• Consuming a diet rich in high-glycemic-index (GI) foods, such as refined carbohydrates (white bread, sugary snacks, and cereals), may contribute to acne development.

• High-GI foods can lead to an increase in insulin levels, which may stimulate sebum production and contribute to inflammation.

Dairy Products:

• Some studies have suggested a potential link between the consumption of dairy products, particularly skim milk, and an increased risk of acne.

Hormones and growth factors in milk may influence skin health.

Omega-6 Fatty Acids:

• An imbalance between omega-6 and omega-3 fatty acids in the diet may contribute to inflammation, which plays a role in acne development.

• Western diets often contain a higher ratio of omega-6 to omega-3 fatty acids.

Antioxidants and Nutrients:

• Inadequate intake of certain nutrients, such as zinc, vitamin E, and vitamin A, may be associated with acne.

Antioxidants play a role in skin health and may help reduce inflammation.

Chocolate and Sweets:

• Some studies have explored a potential association between chocolate consumption and acne.

The link is not universally agreed upon, and more research is needed to establish a clear connection.

It's important to note that individual responses to dietary factors vary, and not everyone will experience the same effects. Additionally, factors like genetics, hormonal changes, and environmental influences also play significant roles in acne development.

While there is evidence suggesting a potential impact of diet on acne, it's crucial to approach this relationship with caution. More research is needed to establish specific dietary guidelines for acne prevention or management. If you suspect that your acne may be influenced by your diet, take into account the following:

Maintain a food journal to track your dietary intake and identify any recurring trends that may indicate a connection between particular foods and acne outbreaks.

It is advisable to implement dietary changes in a gradual manner. Unpredictable alterations might fail to offer definitive insights into the consequences for one's skin.

Seeking Professional Advice: For personalized guidance regarding concerns regarding the correlation between your diet and acne, it is advisable to consult with a dermatologist or other healthcare professional.

Overall, maintaining a balanced diet, staying hydrated, and

practicing good skincare habits are
important components of overall
skin health.

CHAPTER FOUR
Nutrients for Clear Skin

Maintaining a healthy and balanced diet can contribute to clear and radiant skin. While individual responses to nutrients may vary, incorporating certain vitamins, minerals, and other nutrients into your diet can support skin health. Here are some nutrients that are commonly associated with promoting clear skin:

Vitamin A:

• Plays a crucial role in skin health and is essential for the maintenance of healthy skin tissues.

Found in foods like sweet potatoes, carrots, spinach, kale, and liver.

C vitamins:

• Acts as an antioxidant, helping to protect the skin from oxidative stress.

• Promotes collagen production and helps maintain skin elasticity.

Found in citrus fruits, strawberries, bell peppers, and broccoli.

Vitamin E:

• Another antioxidant that helps protect the skin from damage caused by free radicals.

Found in nuts, seeds, spinach, and avocado.

Zinc:

• Supports the immune system and may help reduce inflammation associated with acne.

Found in foods like lean meats, seafood, nuts, and seeds.

The Fatty Acid Omega-3:

• Possess anti-inflammatory properties that may benefit skin health.

Found in fatty fish (salmon, mackerel, sardines), flaxseeds, chia seeds, and walnuts.

Probiotics include:

• Promote a healthy gut microbiome, which is linked to overall well-being, including skin health.

• Found in fermented foods like yogurt, kefir, sauerkraut, and kimchi.

Water:

• Staying well-hydrated is crucial for maintaining skin moisture and supporting overall skin health.

The Element Selenium:

• Antioxidants that may help protect the skin from UV damage.

Found in Brazil nuts, fish, poultry, and whole grains.

Collagen:

• While not a nutrient, collagen is a protein that plays a key role in skin structure and elasticity.

• Collagen-rich foods include bone broth, chicken skin, and fish.

Green Tea:

• Contains antioxidants and anti-inflammatory compounds that may benefit skin health.

It's important to note that while a healthy diet can contribute to clear skin, individual factors, such as genetics, hormones, and skincare habits, also play significant roles. Additionally, if you have specific concerns about your skin or are considering dietary changes for skin health, it's advisable to consult with a dermatologist or a registered dietitian for personalized advice.

Remember that adopting a well-rounded and varied diet, along with good skincare practices, can contribute to overall skin health and clarity.

Antioxidants and Their Role

Antioxidants are compounds that play a crucial role in protecting the body's cells from damage caused by free radicals. Free radicals are unstable molecules produced during normal cellular processes or in response to factors like pollution, UV radiation, and certain lifestyle choices such as smoking. When free radicals accumulate, they can contribute to oxidative stress, which may damage cells, proteins, and DNA, potentially leading to various health issues, including skin problems.

Antioxidants neutralize free radicals by donating electrons, thereby reducing their harmful effects. In the context of skin health, antioxidants are particularly beneficial due to their ability to combat oxidative stress and support overall skin well-being. Here are some common antioxidants and their roles:

Vitamin C (Ascorbic Acid):

Acts As A Powerful Antioxidant.

• Protects the skin from free radicals and supports collagen synthesis.

Found in citrus fruits, strawberries, bell peppers, and broccoli.

Vitamin E (Tocopherol):

• A fat-soluble antioxidant that protects cell membranes from damage.

Found in nuts, seeds, spinach, and vegetable oils.

Beta-Carotene (Provitamin A):

• Converted into vitamin A in the body, playing a role in skin health.

Found in carrots, sweet potatoes, kale, and spinach.

The Element Selenium:

• An essential trace element with antioxidant properties.

• Helps protect the skin from oxidative damage.

Found in Brazil nuts, fish, poultry, and whole grains.

Zinc:

• An essential mineral with antioxidant properties.

• Supports wound healing and immune function.

Found in foods like oysters, beef, and pumpkin seeds.

Polyphenols:

• Found in various plant-based foods, such as green tea, berries, and dark chocolate.

Have antioxidant and anti-inflammatory properties.

Coenzyme Q10 (CoQ10):

• Naturally present in the body, CoQ10 functions as an antioxidant.

• Helps protect skin cells from oxidative stress.

Found in small amounts in some foods and available in supplement form.

Flavonoids:

A group of plant compounds with antioxidant effects.

Found in fruits, vegetables, tea, and red wine.

Astaxanthin:

• A carotenoid with potent antioxidant properties.

Found in microalgae, salmon, shrimp, and krill oil.

Glutathione:

• A potent antioxidant produced in the body.

Supports the detoxification process and helps neutralize free radicals.

In skincare, antioxidants are often incorporated into products to safeguard the skin from environmental damage and promote a healthy complexion. Additionally, consuming a diet abundant in antioxidants can contribute to overall skin health by providing protection from oxidative stress. However, it's crucial to maintain a balanced diet with a variety of nutrient-rich foods for optimal skin benefits. If you have specific skin concerns, consulting with a dermatologist can help guide you toward effective hygiene practices and potential dietary adjustments.

Minerals for Acne Prevention

Certain minerals play essential roles in skin health and may contribute to acne prevention. Here are some minerals that are associated with maintaining healthy skin and may have a role in preventing or managing acne:

Zinc:

• Role in Acne Prevention: Zinc is known for its anti-inflammatory properties and its ability to regulate sebaceous (oil) production. It may help reduce inflammation and prevent congested pores.

Food Sources: Oysters, beef, chicken, pumpkin seeds, and cashews.

The element selenium:

• Role in Acne Prevention: Selenium is an antioxidant that helps safeguard the skin from oxidative stress. It may support overall epidermis health.

Food Sources: Brazil nuts, fish, poultry, whole cereals.

Copper:

• Role in Acne Prevention: Copper is involved in collagen formation, which is crucial for skin structure. It may contribute to overall epidermis health.

Food Sources: Shellfish, liver, almonds, seeds, legumes.

The element magnesium:

Role in Acne Prevention: Magnesium has anti-inflammatory properties and may help regulate hormonal homeostasis, potentially influencing acne development.

Food Sources: Leafy green vegetables, nuts, seeds, whole cereals.

Sulfur:

• Role in Acne Prevention: Sulfur is a component of keratin, which is essential for skin health. It may help promote healthy skin and prevent acne lesions.

Food Sources: Garlic, onions, cruciferous vegetables (broccoli, cabbage).

Silicon:

• Role in Acne Prevention: Silicon is involved in collagen synthesis and connective tissue health, which may support overall skin integrity.

Food Sources: Whole cereals, oats, bananas, seafood.

Iron:

• Role in Acne Prevention: Iron is essential for transporting oxygen to skin cells, supporting their health.

Food Sources: Red meat, poultry, fish, lentils, legumes.

While these minerals may play roles in supporting skin health, it's essential to emphasize that a balanced and varied diet is crucial for overall well-being. Additionally, individual responses to dietary changes can vary, and minerals alone may not be a sole solution for preventing or managing acne.

If you are concerned about acne or skin health, it's recommended to consult with a dermatologist. They can provide personalized advice based on your specific skin type, condition, and lifestyle factors. Skincare routines, hydration, and other lifestyle factors also contribute significantly to overall skin health.

CHAPTER FIVE
Foods to Include for Clear Skin

Including a diversity of nutrient-rich foods in your diet can contribute to clear and healthy skin. While individual responses to dietary changes can range, here are some foods that are generally associated with promoting clear skin:

Fruits and Vegetables:

• Rich in vitamins, minerals, and antioxidants that support skin health.

Include a variety of colorful fruits and vegetables like berries, citrus, leafy greens, carrots, and bell peppers.

Fatty Fish:

• Omega-3 fatty acids found in fish like salmon, mackerel, and sardines have anti-inflammatory properties and may help maintain skin health.

Nuts and Seeds:

• Almonds, walnuts, chia seeds, and flaxseeds provide healthful fats, vitamins, and minerals that support skin function.

Whole Grains:

• Foods like brown rice, quinoa, and oats contain complex

carbohydrates and fiber, fostering stable blood sugar levels, which may be beneficial for acne prevention.

Probiotic-Rich Foods:

• Fermented foods like yogurt, kefir, sauerkraut, and kimchi contain probiotics that support a healthy intestinal microbiome, which can impact skin health.

Lean Proteins:

• Skin-friendly proteins include poultry, fish, tofu, and legumes. Protein is essential for collagen production and overall skin structure.

Water:

• Staying hydrated is crucial for skin health. Water helps flush out toxins and maintains the skin hydrated and supple.

Green Tea:

• Contains antioxidants, notably catechins, which may have anti-inflammatory effects on the skin.

Sweet Potatoes:

• High in beta-carotene, which is converted to vitamin A in the body, supporting skin health.

Avocado:

• Contains healthful monounsaturated fats, vitamin E, and other nutrients that can contribute to smooth and radiant skin.

Bell Peppers:

• High in vitamin C, an antioxidant that supports collagen production and protects the epidermis from oxidative stress.

Dark Chocolate (in moderation):

• High-quality dark chocolate with at least 70% cocoa content contains antioxidants that may benefit the epidermis.

Remember that maintaining clear skin involves a combination of factors, including a balanced diet, appropriate hydration, a consistent skincare routine, and other lifestyle choices. Additionally, individual responses to specific foods can vary, so it's essential to pay attention to how your body reacts to different dietary adjustments. If you have specific concerns about your skin, consulting with a dermatologist can provide personalized advice based on your skin type and condition.

Foods to Avoid for Acne-Free Skin

While individual responses to specific foods can vary, some people may find that certain dietary choices can exacerbate or provoke acne. It's crucial to note that the relationship between diet and acne is still an area of ongoing research, and not everyone will experience the same effects. However, if you're seeking to promote acne-free skin, you may consider minimizing or avoiding the following:

High-Glycemic Foods:

• Foods that rapidly elevate blood sugar levels may contribute to increased insulin production, leading to higher sebum (oil) production. This can potentially contribute to acne.

• Examples include white bread, sugary cereals, confectionery, and pastries.

Dairy Products:

• Some studies suggest a potential association between dairy consumption, particularly skim milk, and an increased risk of acne.

• Consider reducing intake of milk, cheese, and other dairy products.

Chocolate and Sweets:

• While the direct link is not completely established, some studies have explored associations between chocolate consumption and acne.

• Excessive consumption of high-sugar treats may contribute to inflammation and skin issues.

Fast Food and Processed Foods:

• High levels of unhealthy fats, preservatives, and additives found in many fast foods and processed treats may contribute to inflammation and negatively impact skin health.

Fried and Greasy Foods:

• Some individuals find that a diet high in fried and greasy foods is associated with acne breakouts.

• Limiting the ingestion of fried foods and opting for healthier cooking methods may be beneficial.

Excessive Caffeine:

• While moderate caffeine intake is generally considered safe, excessive consumption of caffeinated beverages, especially sweetened ones, may contribute to inflammation.

Alcohol:

• Excessive alcohol consumption can dehydrate the epidermis, potentially leading to an overproduction of oil to compensate.

• Alcohol may also affect the body's inflammatory response.

Iodine-Rich Foods:

• Some studies suggest that excessive iodine intake may exacerbate acne in certain individuals.

Foods abundant in iodine include seaweed, iodized salt, and certain seafood.

Processed Meats:

• Processed meats may contain additives and preservatives that can contribute to inflammation.

• Opt for lean, unprocessed protein sources like poultry, fish, and legumes.

Spicy Foods:

• For some individuals, spicy foods may induce or worsen acne.

Pay attention to how your epidermis responds to spicy meals and adjust accordingly.

It's important to recognize that everyone's skin is unique, and what works for one person may not work for another. If you suspect that your diet is influencing your acne, consider maintaining a food diary to identify potential triggers. A dermatologist can also offer individualized recommendations tailored to your particular skin type and condition.

Prominent Causes of Acne Outbreaks

A variety of factors can contribute to acne flare-ups; therefore, identifying frequent perpetrators can aid in the prevention and management of outbreaks. Although there may be some variation in individual reactions, the following factors frequently contribute to acne flare-ups:

Hormonal Variations:

• Particularly during puberty, menstruation, pregnancy, and hormonal disorders, hormonal fluctuations can stimulate the activity of sebaceous glands, resulting in acne and increased oil production.

Products for Cosmetics and Skincare:

• As a contributor to acne, specific cosmetics and hygiene products may contain substances that clog pores or irritate the skin.

Opt for products that are oil-free and non-comedogenic.

Intestinal Factors:

• Foods with high glycemic index: Sugary and refined carbohydrate-rich foods have the potential to affect insulin levels, which could lead to an increase in the production of sebum.

Some research indicates that the consumption of dairy products may contribute to acne in certain individuals.

The Strain:

• The secretion of hormones such as cortisol in response to stress can promote the generation of sebum and exacerbate episodes of acne.

Inadequate Skincare Practices:

• Excessive bathing or vigorous scrubbing may cause skin irritation and disturb its inherent equilibrium.

The use of pore-clogging or comedogenic products may exacerbate acne.

Pharmaceutical Agents:

• As a side effect, certain medications, such as contraceptives, steroids, and certain anticonvulsants, may contribute to acne.

Environmental Aspects:

• Certain climates, pollution, and humidity can diminish the health of the skin and contribute to the development of acne.

The Study Of Genetics:

• A predisposition to acne may be influenced by an individual's family history.

Bacterial Aspects:

• The presence of Propionibacterium acnes (P. acnes) bacteria on the epidermis may be a factor in acne and inflammation.

The following are pore-clogging ingredients:

• Certain oils and silicones, among other components of hygiene and cosmetic products, may exacerbate the symptoms of acne and clogged pores.

The following are haircare products:

• Migration of haircare products onto the face, particularly those featuring oily or heavy formulations, has the potential to exacerbate acne lesions along the hairline and temples.

Acne can be managed by identifying and targeting particular triggers. Important elements of acne management include adhering to a balanced diet, selecting suitable cosmetics and skincare products, managing stress, and maintaining a consistent and mild skincare routine. In cases of persistent or severe acne, seeking the expertise of a dermatologist can yield customized recommendations and treatment alternatives that are specifically designed to address the individual's condition.

CHAPTER SIX
Developing a Meal Plan for Clear Skin

A meal plan designed to promote clear skin should include an assortment of nutrient-dense foods that are beneficial to the health of the skin. Although diet in isolation may not provide a comprehensive remedy for acne, adhering to a balanced and nutritious diet can positively impact one's overall health, including that of the skin. A sample meal schedule for clear skin is as follows:

For breakfast,

• Oats cooked overnight with a combination of chia seeds, fruit, and a garnish of pumpkin seeds.

Hydrogen or green tea.

The midmorning snack consists of:

• A drizzle of honey accompanied by a fistful of almonds and Greek yogurt.

A portion of freshly harvested produce, such as a handful of berries or an apple.

Dish for Lunch:

• Tofu or grilled chicken salad comprised of avocado, cucumbers, cherry tomatoes, and assorted greens.

Sides of brown rice or quinoa.

Tahini and lemon vinaigrette.

Purée of herbs or water.

Snack to Follow:

• Cucumber and carrot skewers spread with hummus.

A fistful of sunflower seeds or walnuts.

Meal: Dinner

• Salmon that has been baked or a plant-based protein alternative (such as legumes or lentils).

• Broccoli and sweet potatoes that are roasted.

Mixed leafy greens dressed with citrus and olive oil as a side dish.

Purée of herbs or water.

Snack in the evening (optional):

• A small serving of assorted berries or a piece of dark chocolate containing a minimum of 70% cocoa.

Sufficient hydration:

• Drink copious amounts of water throughout the day. Maintaining adequate hydration is vital for healthy, clear skin.

Aspects to Consider:

• **Omega-3 oily Acids:** The omega-3 content of oily fish (salmon, mackerel), chia seeds, and flaxseeds may have anti-inflammatory properties.

Consume a diverse assortment of vibrant fruits and vegetables to augment your intake of antioxidants, which are known to promote optimal skin condition.

Lean protein sources, such as chicken, fish, tofu, and legumes, assist in the promotion of collagen synthesis and the maintenance of optimal skin structure.

Opt for whole grains such as quinoa and brown rice in order to obtain fiber and complex carbohydrates, both of which contribute to blood sugar regulation.

Greek yogurt, kefir, and other fermented foods are examples of probiotic foods that may influence skin health by promoting a healthy intestinal microbiome.

Bear in mind that individual reactions to dietary modifications differ, and it is critical to monitor your body's reaction to various foods. For individuals with particular dietary restrictions or complexion concerns, seeking advice from a registered dietitian or a healthcare professional can offer tailored recommendations. Furthermore, in order to attain and sustain clear skin, it is critical to attend to stress management, adequate sleep, and proper hygiene regimens.

Optimizing Nutrient Balance for Optimal Impact

Maintaining a nutrient balance in one's diet is critical for overall health, which includes the promotion of clear, healthy skin. For optimal results when it comes to balancing nutrients on the epidermis, consider the following:

Consist Of An Assortment Of Nutrient-Dense Foods:

• To ensure a comprehensive array of nutrients, strive to incorporate a variety of fruits, vegetables, whole cereals, lean proteins, and healthy fats into your diet.

Balance of Omega-3 and Omega-6:

• To offset the prevalence of omega-6 fatty acids in vegetable oils, integrate omega-3 fatty acid sources (fatty fish, chia seeds, flaxseeds). A balanced proportion can aid in the reduction of inflammation.

Strengthen Antioxidants:

• Protect the epidermis against oxidative stress by incorporating an assortment of foods that are abundant in antioxidants, including but not limited to berries, citrus fruits, leafy greens, and nuts.

Protein Consumption:

• It is imperative to consume a sufficient quantity of lean proteins, such as those found in poultry, fish, tofu, and legumes, in order to promote collagen synthesis and maintain optimal skin structure.

Consistent Carbohydrates:

• By restricting refined carbohydrates and opting for complex carbohydrates derived from whole grains (quinoa, brown rice), individuals can potentially mitigate the risk of acne by promoting blood sugar stability.

Beneficial Fats:

• Include healthful fat sources in your diet, such as avocados, nuts, seeds, and olive oil. These lipids play a vital role in preserving the integrity of the skin barrier.

Sufficient hydration:

• To maintain proper hydration, consume copious amounts of water throughout the day. Constant hydration is critical for preserving the moisture of the epidermis and promoting its overall health.

Practicing Mindful Eating:

• Pay heed to the hunger and satiety cues your body sends. By cultivating the practice of mindful dining, one can nurture a positive and balanced relationship with food.

The Difference Between Probiotics and Prebiotics:

• Promoting skin health is the consumption of probiotic-rich foods (yogurt, kefir, fermented foods), which help maintain a healthy intestinal microbiome. Additionally, prebiotic foods (such as garlic, onions, and bananas) support beneficial gut flora.

Minerals and vitamins:

• Ensure sufficient consumption of vital vitamins and minerals that are integral to skin health, such as selenium, zinc, A, C, and E.

Restrict Possible Triggers:

• If you have observed that certain foods elicit skin problems, you may wish to decrease your consumption of those foods while following your skin's reaction.

Bear in mind that individual reactions to dietary modifications may differ. For individualized guidance regarding epidermis concerns or dietary requirements, it is advisable to seek the opinion of a registered dietitian or another healthcare professional. In addition, cultivating a harmonious lifestyle, adhering to effective skincare routines, effectively managing tension, and ensuring adequate sleep are essential elements in the promotion of radiant and healthy skin.

CHAPTER SEVEN
Habits of Lifestyle for Clear Skin

Certain lifestyle choices can complement a well-balanced hygiene regimen and a nutritious diet to promote clear, healthy skin. The following lifestyle choices can aid in the attainment and preservation of clear skin:

Sufficient hydration:

• Throughout the day, consume copious amounts of water to hydrate the epidermis and flush out toxins. Adequate hydration is essential for maintaining skin elasticity and a clear complexion.

Consistent Exercise:

• Circulation is improved through regular physical activity, which can aid in the transportation of nutrients and oxygen to the epidermis cells. Additionally, stress reduction facilitated by exercise can contribute to clearer complexion.

Sufficient Sleep:

• Allocate sufficient quality sleep on a nightly basis to facilitate bodily repair and regeneration. Insomnia has the potential to induce heightened levels of tension and inflammation, both of which can worsen skin conditions.

Stress Administration:

• Engage in practices that alleviate tension, such as yoga, meditation, deep breathing, or mindfulness. Prolonged stress has the potential to induce hormonal disruptions and inflammation, which may exacerbate acne and other dermatological conditions.

Sun Protection Measures:

• Even on overcast days, apply a broad-spectrum sunscreen (SPF 30 or higher) daily. An elevated risk of developing skin cancer, sunburn, and premature aging are all consequences of solar exposure.

Opt for an oil-free, non-comedogenic sunscreen to prevent pore blockage.

Routine Skincare with Care:

• Twice daily, cleanse your skin with a mild cleanser that is appropriate for your skin type. Scrubbing or over-cleansing excessively can cause irritation and disturb the skin's natural equilibrium.

• Utilize hygiene products that do not contain comedogens to prevent pore clogging and acne exacerbation.

Refrain from smoking and consuming alcohol in excess:

While excessive alcohol consumption can dehydrate the skin and worsen skin conditions such as rosacea and acne, smoking can hasten the aging process and hinder the recovery of the skin.

Consistent Skin Examinations:

• Consistently inspect your skin for any modifications, including the development of new moles, lesions, or irregularities. Detection of cutaneous conditions in their early stages enables prompt intervention and treatment.

Promoting Positive Relationships and Social Interactions:

• Develop relationships of support and participate in social activities that bring you happiness. Additionally, positive social interactions can promote skin health and overall well-being by reducing stress.

Refrain from touching your face:

• Restrictive facial touching and plucking can promote the proliferation of bacteria, skin irritation, and subsequent occurrences of acne or inflammation.

Environmental Factor Management:

• By utilizing barrier creams and moisturizing or windproofing products, you can shield your skin from severe environmental conditions such as extreme cold or wind.

• Restrict one's exposure to toxins and environmental pollutants that are known to cause inflammation and skin injury.

By integrating these lifestyle practices into one's daily regimen, one can internally promote clear and healthy skin. Bear in mind the importance of consistency, and it might require some time to observe discernible progress. For individuals with particularized inquiries or skin-related concerns, it is advisable to seek the guidance of a dermatologist or skincare expert.

The Value of Consistent Exercise

Consistent physical activity is essential for optimal health and well-being, as it imparts advantages to multiple facets of mental, emotional, and physical health. Key reasons emphasizing the significance of regular exercise include the following:

Health of the Cardiovascular System:

• By enhancing circulation and fortifying the heart, regular exercise reduces the risk of cardiovascular diseases like heart attacks and strokes.

The Management of Weight:

• Active engagement in physical activity is crucial for weight maintenance as it facilitates the combustion of calories and the promotion of fat loss. It also prevents conditions associated with obesity.

Bone and Muscle Health:

• By promoting the development and maintenance of robust bones and muscles, weight-bearing exercises and resistance training reduce the risk of osteoporosis and frailty.

Strengthened Mental Health:

• Engaging in physical activity has been associated with a decreased likelihood of developing depression and anxiety. Engagement in physical activity elicits the secretion of endorphins, commonly referred to as "feel-good" hormones, which elevate mood.

Enhanced Function of the Mind:

• Engaging in consistent physical activity has been linked to enhanced cognitive abilities, such as improved memory, concentration, and learning.

Improved Sleep:

• Regular physical activity can assist in the regulation of sleep patterns and the enhancement of sleep quality. Nevertheless, the impacts of engaging in vigorous exercise near nighttime can differ among individuals.

Stress Mitigation:

• Stress can be effectively managed through physical activity, which decreases cortisol levels and induces relaxation. It affords the chance to cleanse the mind and concentrate on the present.

Increased Levels of Energy:

• Consistent engagement in physical exercise contributes to an overall increase in energy and stamina. It enhances cardiovascular efficacy, thereby reducing the perceived exertion of routine activities.

Strengthened Immune System:

• A strengthened immune system has been associated with moderate, consistent exercise, which reduces the risk of illness and promotes overall health.

Social Communication:

• Participating in group exercises or team athletics facilitates social interaction, thereby cultivating a sense of community and camaraderie.

Mitigated Risk of Chronic Illnesses:

• Consistent physical activity is correlated with a reduced likelihood of developing chronic ailments, including metabolic syndrome, type 2 diabetes, and specific forms of cancer.

Body Image and Self-Esteem Enhancement:

• The attainment of fitness objectives and the enjoyment of the physical advantages of exercise can positively influence an individual's self-perception and self-worth.

The concept of longevity:

• There is a correlation between an active lifestyle and increased longevity. It has been demonstrated that consistent physical activity prolongs life and healthful aging.

Notably, individual preferences, health conditions, and fitness levels can influence both the nature and intensity of physical activity. It is prudent for individuals with pre-existing health conditions to seek guidance from a healthcare professional or fitness expert prior to commencing a new exercise regimen in order to ascertain its suitability and safety. A balanced regimen comprising aerobic exercises, strength training, and flexibility activities has the potential to yield numerous health advantages.

Methods to Achieve Clear Skin

Although precise recipes cannot ensure flawless skin, integrating ingredients that are abundant in nutrients into one's diet can positively impact the overall health of the skin. The following are two recipes that highlight ingredients recognized for their potential skin benefits:

- Salmon and Quinoa Bowl (Recipe 1)
- The following are ingredients:
- Cup quinoa, heated
- Salmon fillet, 6 ounces, broiled or grilled
- One cup of arugula, spinach, or kale, in a mixed salad
- 1/2 diced avocado
- 1/4 cup halved cherry tomatoes
- 1 tablespoon olive oil, extra-virgin
- In place of lemon segments as a garnish
- Pepper and salt to flavor

Means of instruction:

- Cook quinoa per the instructions on the package.

- After seasoning the salmon fillet with pepper and salt, bake or grill it until thoroughly cooked.

- Combine cooked quinoa, assorted greens, avocado slices, and cherry tomatoes in a bowl.

- On top, arrange the seared salmon.

- Squeeze fresh lemon juice over the bowl, drizzle with extra-virgin olive oil, and season to flavor with salt and pepper.

- Bowl of Berry Smoothies (Recipe 2)

The Following Are Ingredients:

- 1 cup berry mixture (including strawberries, blueberries, and raspberries)
- Frozen banana, half
- Half cup yogurt made with Greek yogurt
- 1 teaspoonful of chia flour
- 1 teaspoonful buttery almonds
- One-fourth cup cereals
- Drizzling honey is optional.

- Means of instruction:

- Smoothly blend the frozen banana, assorted berries, Greek yogurt, chia seeds, and almond butter.

- The smoothie is poured into a dish.

- Plating should include granola and, if preferred, honey drizzle.

Note: The ingredients in these recipes are abundant in vitamins, minerals, antioxidants, and omega-3 fatty acids, all of which may be advantageous to the complexion. Nevertheless, individual reactions to these components might differ, and it is critical to uphold a well-rounded dietary regimen.

Bear in mind that a radiant and sound complexion is impacted by a multitude of elements, encompassing holistic nourishment, sufficient hydration, hygiene routines, and lifestyle decisions. For individuals with particularized inquiries regarding their epidermis health, it is advisable to seek personalized guidance from a registered dietitian or dermatologist.

Supplements to Heal Acne

Although a well-rounded diet loaded with vital nutrients is imperative for general well-being and may positively impact skin health, exercising prudence is advised when considering the use of supplements to aid in the healing of acne. Before adding any new supplements to your routine, it is vital to consult a healthcare professional, as individual requirements vary and excessive use of certain supplements may cause adverse effects.

However, certain dietary supplements have been

investigated for their potential efficacy in acne treatment and skin health support. The following have been investigated:

Zinc:

• Due to its involvement in wound healing and immune function, zinc may aid in the reduction of acne-related inflammation. Zinc is offered as a dietary supplement; however, overconsumption may result in toxicity; therefore, it is critical to seek guidance from a healthcare professional regarding the correct dosage.

The Fatty Acid Omega-3:

• Omega-3 fatty acids, which are present in fish oil supplements, potentially promote skin health and possess anti-inflammatory properties. It is advisable to seek guidance from a healthcare professional regarding the appropriate dosage and to verify that it is compatible with your overall health.

Vitamin A:

• Vitamin A influences skin health, and for severe acne, isotretinoin, a vitamin A derivative, is sometimes prescribed. Nevertheless, an overabundance of vitamin A may result in toxicity. Before contemplating supplements, it is vital to obtain vitamin A from dietary sources and consult a healthcare professional.

Probiotics include:

• Supplemental probiotics comprise advantageous microorganisms that promote gut health. A number of studies indicate the possibility of a connection between gastrointestinal health and skin disorders, such as acne. Although probiotics are available in supplement form and fermented foods, their efficacy in treating acne is still the subject of ongoing research.

Vitamin D:

• Although vitamin D is critical for immune function, its potential impact on cutaneous health has been the subject of some research. However, vitamin D can be detrimental in excess; therefore, it is best to obtain vitamin D from food and sunlight, or consult a healthcare professional before taking supplements.

It is imperative to underscore the fact that supplements ought not to supplant a diverse and well-balanced diet. Obtaining nutrients from whole foods is frequently preferable to supplementation with isolated substances. If you are contemplating the use of dietary supplements for acne or have concerns about the potential deficiency of specific nutrients in your diet, it is advisable to seek personalized guidance from a healthcare professional, preferable a registered dietitian or dermatologist, in accordance with your unique health condition.

It is important to consider the substantial influence of lifestyle factors, hygiene routines, and adequate hydration on acne management. Frequently, adopting a holistic approach yields the most favorable results.

Conclusion

In summary, the attainment and sustenance of flawless and robust skin necessitate a comprehensive strategy encompassing adjustments to one's nutrition, skincare routine, way of life, and, if required, consultation with healthcare experts. Here are several important takeaways:

• A well-balanced diet, which comprises an abundance of nutrient-dense foods such as fruits, vegetables, lean proteins, and healthy lipids, has the potential to promote skin clarity and enhance overall health. Skin health requires essential nutrients such as vitamins, minerals, antioxidants, and omega-3 fatty acids.

• **Hygiene Routine:** It is essential to maintain healthy skin by establishing a gentle and consistent hygiene routine. It is advisable to utilize products that are appropriate for one's skin type and to refrain from using harsh chemicals that have the potential to irritate or obstruct pores. Consistent sun protection, cleansing, and moisturizing are vital components.

Adopting healthy lifestyle practices, including consistent physical activity, sufficient rest, effective stress management, and sufficient hydration, can have a beneficial effect on the condition of one's skin. These behaviors enhance general health and potentially aid in the prevention or treatment of skin disorders.

- **Supplements:** Although certain supplements have been investigated for their potential efficacy in promoting skin health and treating acne, it is crucial to seek guidance from healthcare professionals prior to integrating them into one's regimen. Certain dietary supplements may cause adverse effects when consumed in excess.

• **Individual Variability:** Due to the fact that each person is distinct, reactions to modifications in diet, hygiene regimen, and way of life may differ. Time may be required to determine the most efficacious method for addressing your particular skin concerns.

It is recommended that individuals with persistent or severe skin concerns consult healthcare professionals, including registered dietitians or dermatologists, for guidance and recommendations. Given your unique skin type, condition, and general health, they are capable of offering customized recommendations and treatment alternatives.

Bear in mind that clear skin frequently serves as an indicator of holistic health and well-being. Embracing a holistic perspective that takes into account multiple determinants may enhance one's complexion and overall state of wellness. Consistently monitoring your skin in conjunction with an informed and proactive hygiene regimen will assist you in attaining and sustaining optimal skin health.

THE END